I0765454

ABRAXXZAS

ONIONOMICS

Unlocking Nature's Health Secret

First published by Okam Kalu 2024

Copyright © 2024 by Abraxxzas

All rights reserved. No part of this publication may be reproduced, stored or transmitted in any form or by any means, electronic, mechanical, photocopying, recording, scanning, or otherwise without written permission from the publisher. It is illegal to copy this book, post it to a website, or distribute it by any other means without permission.

Abraxxzas asserts the moral right to be identified as the author of this work.

Abraxxzas has no responsibility for the persistence or accuracy of URLs for external or third-party Internet Websites referred to in this publication and does not guarantee that any content on such Websites is, or will remain, accurate or appropriate.

Designations used by companies to distinguish their products are often claimed as trademarks. All brand names and product names used in this book and on its cover are trade names, service marks, trademarks and registered trademarks of their respective owners. The publishers and the book are not associated with any product or vendor mentioned in this book. None of the companies referenced within the book have endorsed the book.

First edition

This book was professionally typeset on Reedsy.
Find out more at reedsy.com

Contents

1

Chapter 1

"Life is like an onion: You peel it off one layer at a time, and sometimes you weep." - Carl Sandburg

3

ONIONOMICS

4

Unlocking Nature's Health Secret

5

Chapter 1: The Humble Onion: An Introduction

In the realm of culinary delights and nutritional powerhouses, the humble onion stands as a stalwart champion. With its unassuming appearance and ubiquitous presence in kitchens around the world, the onion often goes unrecognized for its remarkable health benefits and culinary versatility. Yet, beneath its unassuming layers lies a treasure trove of nutrients, antioxidants, and medicinal properties waiting to be discovered.

For centuries, onions have been a staple ingredient in countless cuisines, valued not only for their unique flavor but also for their ability to enhance the taste of dishes in diverse culinary traditions. Whether sliced, diced, or caramelized, onions add depth and complexity to soups, stews, salads, and stir-fries, elevating ordinary meals to extraordinary culinary experiences.

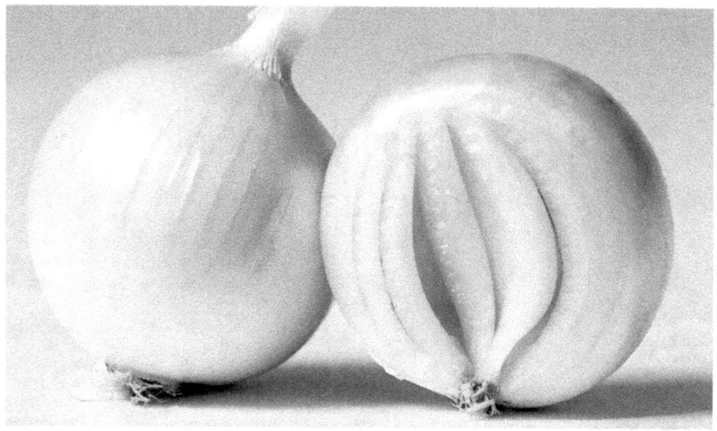

But beyond their culinary allure, onions possess a wealth of health-promoting properties that have been celebrated since ancient times. From boosting immunity to supporting heart health, onions have earned their status as a true superfood, revered for their medicinal qualities as much as their culinary appeal.

In this journey through the world of onions, we will explore the rich history, nutritional composition, and health benefits of this unassuming vegetable. We will delve into the science behind its therapeutic effects, uncovering the secrets that make onions a potent ally in the quest for wellness.

Join me as we peel back the layers of mystery surrounding the onion and unlock the secrets of its remarkable health-promoting properties. Together, we will embark on a journey of discovery, celebrating the extraordinary potential hidden within nature's humble treasure: the onion.

Chapter 2: A Brief History of Onions

From the ancient civilizations of Mesopotamia and Egypt to the bustling markets of modern-day cities, the onion has traversed both time and space, leaving an indelible mark on human history. Its journey is as storied as it is ancient, intertwined with the evolution of human culture, trade, and culinary traditions.

The origins of the onion can be traced back thousands of years, with archaeological evidence suggesting that it was cultivated as early as 5000 BCE in the region of present-day Iran and Pakistan. From there, its cultivation spread across ancient civilizations, including the Sumerians, Babylonians, and Egyptians, who revered the onion for its culinary and medicinal properties.

In ancient Egypt, onions held such significance that they were used as currency, and were placed in the tombs of pharaohs as offerings for the afterlife. The workers who built the Great Pyramid of Giza were said to have been fed onions to keep them strong and healthy, attesting to the vegetable's esteemed status in Egyptian society.

The Greeks and Romans also embraced the onion, both as a culinary ingredient and as a symbol of strength and endurance. Greek athletes consumed onions before competing in the Olympic Games, believing that they imparted stamina and courage. Meanwhile, the Roman legions carried onions with them on their conquests, recognizing their value not only as food but also as a source of sustenance during long campaigns.

As trade routes expanded and civilizations flourished, the onion found its way into the culinary traditions of cultures around the world. In Asia, onions became integral to the cuisines of countries like India, China, and Thailand, adding depth and flavor to a diverse array of dishes. In Europe, onions were embraced by medieval cooks and featured prominently in the recipes of kings and peasants alike.

With the arrival of European settlers in the Americas, onions were introduced to the New World, where they found fertile soil and thrived in a favorable climate. Today, onions are grown on every continent except Antarctica, a testament to their adaptability and enduring popularity.

As we embark on our exploration of onions and their health benefits, let us pause to reflect on the rich tapestry of history that surrounds this humble vegetable. From its humble beginnings in ancient civilizations to its global ubiquity in modern cuisine, the onion has stood the test of time, earning its place as a cherished ingredient in kitchens and cultures around the world.

7

Chapter 3: Varieties of Onions and Their Characteristics

The world of onions is as diverse as it is flavorful, with a wide array of varieties offering unique tastes, textures, and culinary applications. From sweet and mild to pungent and robust, each type of onion brings its distinct character to the table, allowing for endless creativity in the kitchen. In this chapter, we will explore some of the most common varieties of onions and their characteristics.

Yellow Onions:

- Perhaps the most versatile of all onions, yellow onions are widely used in cooking due to their balanced flavor and moderate pungency.
- With a golden-brown skin and white flesh tinged with yellow, these onions develop a rich, sweet flavor when cooked, making them ideal for caramelizing, sautéing, and frying.
- Yellow onions are a staple in savory dishes such as soups, stews, sauces, and casseroles, where their robust flavor adds depth and complexity.

Red Onions:

- Characterized by their vibrant purple skin and crisp, white flesh, red onions are prized for their mild sweetness and striking color.
- Red onions are often enjoyed raw, either sliced thinly in salads, sandwiches, and salsas or pickled for a tangy kick.
- When cooked, red onions retain their color and texture, making them a colorful addition to grilled vegetables, pizzas, and tacos.

White Onions:

- With their ivory-white skin and translucent flesh, white onions offer a mild, slightly sweet flavor that is well-suited to a variety of dishes.
- White onions are commonly used in Mexican and Latin American cuisines, where their delicate flavor complements spicy and tangy ingredients.
- They are often diced and added to salsas, guacamole, and

ceviche, or used to flavor soups, sauces, and marinades.

Sweet Onions:

- True to their name, sweet onions are prized for their high sugar content and mild, sweet flavor, which sets them apart from other varieties.
- Vidalia onions, Walla Walla onions, and Maui onions are popular varieties of sweet onions, each with its own unique taste and growing region.
- Sweet onions are delicious when eaten raw in salads or sandwiches, and they caramelize beautifully when cooked, adding a natural sweetness to dishes like onion rings, French onion soup, and grilled meats.

Shallots:

- Smaller and more elongated than other onions, shallots have a delicate, nuanced flavor that is both sweet and savory.
- Shallots are prized for their ability to add depth and complexity to dishes without overpowering other ingredients, making them a favorite among chefs.
- They are commonly used in French and Mediterranean cuisines, where they are minced and added to dressings, vinaigrettes, sauces, and braises.

As you explore the world of onions, take delight in experimenting with different varieties and discovering the unique flavors they have to offer. Whether you prefer the boldness of yellow onions, the sweetness of red onions, or the delicacy of shallots, there is an onion variety to suit every palate and culinary preference.

13

8

Chapter 4: Nutritional Composition of Onions

In addition to their culinary versatility and distinct flavor profiles, onions boast an impressive array of nutrients that contribute to their status as a nutritional powerhouse. From vitamins and minerals to antioxidants and fiber, onions offer a wide range of health-promoting compounds that support over-all well-being. In this chapter, we will explore the nutritional composition of onions and the benefits they provide.

Vitamins:

- Onions are a good source of several vitamins, including

vitamin C, vitamin B6, and folate.

- Vitamin C is an antioxidant that supports immune function, collagen production, and wound healing.
- Vitamin B6 plays a role in metabolism, brain function, and the formation of red blood cells.
- Folate is essential for DNA synthesis and cell growth, making it particularly important during pregnancy.

Minerals:

- Onions contain various minerals, such as potassium, manganese, and phosphorus.
- Potassium helps regulate blood pressure, fluid balance, and muscle function.
- Manganese is involved in bone formation, metabolism, and antioxidant defense.
- Phosphorus is important for bone health, energy metabolism, and DNA synthesis.

Antioxidants:

- Onions are rich in antioxidants, including flavonoids, polyphenols, and sulfur compounds.
- Quercetin is a powerful antioxidant found in onions that has anti-inflammatory and immune-boosting properties.
- Anthocyanins give red and purple onions their vibrant color and have been linked to heart health and cancer prevention.
- Organosulfur compounds, such as allyl sulfides, contribute to the pungent aroma of onions and have potential anti-cancer effects.

Fiber:

- Onions are a good source of dietary fiber, which supports digestive health and promotes satiety.
- Fiber helps regulate bowel movements, prevent constipation, and reduce the risk of colon cancer.
- Onions contain both soluble and insoluble fiber, which contribute to overall digestive function and may help lower cholesterol levels.

Low in Calories:

- Despite their nutrient density, onions are low in calories, making them a nutritious addition to any diet.
- A half-cup serving of chopped onions contains approximately 30 calories, making them a guilt-free way to add flavor and nutrition to meals.

By incorporating onions into your diet regularly, you can enjoy the nutritional benefits they provide while enhancing the taste and texture of your favorite dishes. Whether raw or cooked, onions are a delicious and nutritious addition to salads, soups, stir-fries, and more, making them a versatile ingredient for culinary exploration.

9

Chapter 5: Antioxidants in Onions: Nature's Defense

In the realm of nutritional superheroes, antioxidants reign supreme, and onions are packed with these powerful compounds that serve as nature's defense against oxidative stress and cellular damage. Antioxidants play a crucial role in maintaining overall health and well-being by neutralizing harmful free radicals and reducing the risk of chronic diseases. In this chapter, we will delve into the abundance of antioxidants found in onions and their remarkable health benefits.

Quercetin:

- Quercetin is a flavonoid antioxidant that is abundant in onions and has been extensively studied for its health-promoting properties.
- As a potent antioxidant and anti-inflammatory agent, quercetin helps protect cells from oxidative damage and reduce inflammation throughout the body.
- Research suggests that quercetin may help lower blood pressure, improve heart health, and reduce the risk of cardiovascular disease by promoting healthy blood flow and reducing cholesterol levels.

Anthocyanins:

- Anthocyanins are another group of antioxidants found in red and purple onions, responsible for their vibrant hues.
- These compounds have been shown to possess strong anti-inflammatory and antioxidant properties, protecting cells from damage caused by free radicals.
- Studies suggest that anthocyanins may help improve cognitive function, support immune health, and reduce the risk of chronic diseases such as cancer and diabetes.

Organosulfur Compounds:

- Onions are rich in organosulfur compounds, which give them their distinctive aroma and flavor.
- These compounds, including diallyl sulfide and allyl propyl disulfide, have been linked to various health benefits, including anticancer effects and immune support.
- Organosulfur compounds have been shown to inhibit the growth of cancer cells, promote detoxification, and enhance

the body's natural defense mechanisms against pathogens and toxins.

Vitamin C:

- While not unique to onions, vitamin C is an essential antioxidant found in abundance in these flavorful bulbs.
- Vitamin C plays a vital role in supporting immune function, collagen synthesis, and wound healing, making it a crucial nutrient for overall health and vitality.
- By neutralizing free radicals and protecting against oxidative damage, vitamin C helps maintain healthy skin, strengthen the immune system, and reduce the risk of chronic diseases such as cancer and heart disease.

Incorporating antioxidant-rich foods like onions into your diet is a simple yet effective way to boost your intake of these health-promoting compounds and support overall well-being. Whether enjoyed raw in salads, sautéed in stir-fries, or caramelized in savory dishes, onions offer a delicious and nutritious way to harness the power of antioxidants and nourish your body from the inside out.

10

Chapter 6: Onions and Heart Health

A healthy heart is the cornerstone of overall well-being, and onions have emerged as a promising ally in the quest for cardiovascular wellness. Packed with an array of heart-friendly nutrients and bioactive compounds, onions offer a natural and flavorful way to support heart health and reduce the risk of cardiovascular disease. In this chapter, we will explore the relationship between onions and heart health, uncovering the mechanisms by which these humble bulbs promote cardiovascular wellness.

Blood Pressure Regulation:

- High blood pressure, or hypertension, is a significant risk factor for heart disease and stroke. Fortunately, onions contain compounds that may help lower blood pressure and promote healthy circulation.
- Quercetin, a potent antioxidant found in onions, has been shown to relax blood vessels, improve endothelial function, and reduce inflammation, all of which contribute to lower blood pressure levels.
- Studies have found that consuming onions regularly may lead to modest reductions in blood pressure, particularly in individuals with hypertension or elevated blood pressure levels.

Cholesterol Management:

- Elevated cholesterol levels, especially LDL cholesterol, can increase the risk of atherosclerosis and heart disease. Fortunately, onions contain compounds that may help lower cholesterol levels and improve lipid profiles.
- Sulfur compounds found in onions, such as allyl sulfides, have been shown to inhibit cholesterol synthesis in the liver and increase the excretion of cholesterol from the body, leading to lower LDL cholesterol levels.
- Additionally, onions contain fiber, particularly soluble fiber, which can help lower cholesterol by binding to cholesterol in the digestive tract and promoting its elimination from the body.

Anti-inflammatory Effects:

- Chronic inflammation is believed to play a significant role in the development of cardiovascular disease. Onions contain anti-inflammatory compounds, such as quercetin and anthocyanins, which may help reduce inflammation and protect against heart disease.

- By neutralizing free radicals and inhibiting inflammatory pathways, these compounds help prevent damage to blood vessels and tissues that can lead to atherosclerosis and heart disease.
- Including onions in a balanced diet rich in other anti-inflammatory foods, such as fruits, vegetables, and whole grains, may help reduce the risk of chronic inflammation and promote heart health.

Antithrombotic Properties:

- Onions possess antithrombotic properties, meaning they can help prevent the formation of blood clots that can lead to heart attacks and strokes.
- Compounds found in onions, including quercetin and sulfur compounds, have been shown to inhibit platelet aggregation and reduce the risk of blood clot formation, particularly in individuals at risk for thrombotic events.

By incorporating onions into your diet regularly, you can enjoy their heart-healthy benefits and support cardiovascular wellness. Whether raw in salads, cooked in soups and stir-fries, or caramelized in savory dishes, onions offer a delicious and nutritious way to nourish your heart and protect against heart disease.

Chapter 7: Onions and Digestive Wellness

A healthy digestive system is essential for overall well-being, and onions have long been valued for their ability to support digestive health and promote optimal digestion. Packed with fiber, prebiotics, and digestive enzymes, onions offer a natural and flavorful way to maintain a happy and healthy gut. In this chapter, we will explore the relationship between onions and digestive wellness, uncovering the mechanisms by which these versatile vegetables promote gastrointestinal health.

Fiber Content:

- Onions are rich in dietary fiber, both soluble and insoluble, which plays a crucial role in supporting digestive health.
- Soluble fiber found in onions helps absorb water and form a gel-like substance in the digestive tract, which aids in softening stools and promoting regular bowel movements.
- Insoluble fiber adds bulk to stool and speeds up transit time through the digestive system, helping prevent constipation and promoting overall digestive regularity.

Prebiotic Properties:

- Onions contain prebiotic fibers, such as inulin and fructooli gosaccharides (FOS), which serve as food for beneficial gut bacteria.
- These prebiotic fibers pass undigested through the upper gastrointestinal tract and reach the colon, where they are fermented by gut bacteria, promoting the growth of beneficial probiotic bacteria.
- By nourishing the gut microbiota, onions help maintain a healthy balance of gut bacteria, support immune function, and protect against digestive disorders such as irritable bowel syndrome (IBS) and inflammatory bowel disease (IBD).

Digestive Enzymes:

- Onions contain natural enzymes, such as amylase and protease, which aid in the digestion of carbohydrates and proteins, respectively.
- These enzymes help break down complex carbohydrates and proteins into simpler molecules that are easier for the

body to absorb and utilize, promoting efficient digestion and nutrient absorption.

- Consuming onions alongside meals can help enhance the digestion of other foods and alleviate symptoms of indigestion, bloating, and discomfort.

Anti-inflammatory Effects:

- Chronic inflammation in the digestive tract can contribute to digestive disorders such as inflammatory bowel disease (IBD) and gastroesophageal reflux disease (GERD).
- Onions possess anti-inflammatory properties, thanks to their rich content of antioxidants such as quercetin and anthocyanins, which help reduce inflammation and protect against oxidative damage in the digestive system.
- By mitigating inflammation, onions may help alleviate symptoms of digestive disorders and promote overall digestive wellness.

Incorporating onions into your diet can be a delicious and effective way to support digestive health and promote overall well-being. Whether raw in salads, cooked in soups and stews, or sautéed in stir-fries, onions offer a versatile and nutritious addition to any meal, providing essential nutrients and digestive support with every bite.

Chapter 8: Onions: A Natural Immune Booster

In an era where immunity is paramount, onions emerge as a potent ally in fortifying the body's natural defenses against illness and infection. Bursting with immune-boosting nutrients and bioactive compounds, onions offer a flavorful and versatile way to support immune health and enhance the body's ability to fend off pathogens. In this chapter, we will explore the role of onions as a natural immune booster and uncover the mechanisms by which they promote immune resilience.

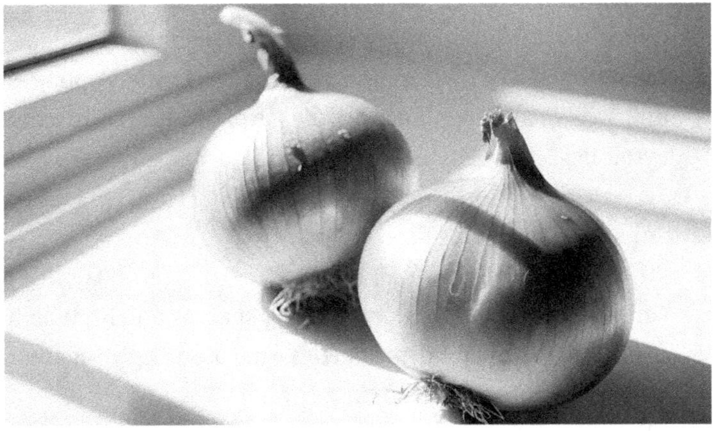

Vitamin C:

- Onions are a good source of vitamin C, a powerful antioxidant that plays a crucial role in supporting immune function.
- Vitamin C enhances the production and function of white blood cells, which are the body's primary defense against infections and pathogens.
- By neutralizing free radicals and reducing oxidative stress, vitamin C helps strengthen the immune system and protect against illness and infection.

Quercetin:

- Quercetin, a flavonoid antioxidant found abundantly in onions, exhibits potent immune-boosting properties.
- Studies have shown that quercetin possesses antiviral, antibacterial, and anti-inflammatory effects, making it effec-

tive at combating a wide range of pathogens.
- Quercetin helps modulate the immune response by enhancing the activity of immune cells, such as macrophages and T cells, and reducing the release of pro-inflammatory cytokines.

Antimicrobial Compounds:

- Onions contain sulfur compounds, such as allicin, which exhibit antimicrobial properties that help fight against bacteria, viruses, and fungi.
- Allicin is released when onions are chopped or crushed, giving them their characteristic pungent odor and potent antimicrobial activity.
- By inhibiting the growth of harmful microorganisms, onions help protect against infections and support overall immune health.

Anti-inflammatory Effects:

- Chronic inflammation can weaken the immune system and increase the risk of illness and disease.
- Onions possess anti-inflammatory properties due to their high content of antioxidants, such as quercetin and anthocyanins, which help reduce inflammation and support immune function.
- By mitigating inflammation, onions help create an environment in the body that is conducive to optimal immune function, allowing the immune system to respond effectively to pathogens and invaders.

Incorporating onions into your diet is a simple yet effective way to bolster your immune defenses and promote overall health and well-being. Whether raw in salads, cooked in soups and stews, or caramelized in savory dishes, onions offer a delicious and nutritious way to support immune resilience and protect against illness and infection.

13

Chapter 9: Onions and Bone Health

While onions may not be commonly associated with bone health, emerging research suggests that these flavorful bulbs contain compounds that can play a role in supporting bone strength and density. With their rich array of nutrients and bioactive compounds, onions offer a unique contribution to skeletal wellness, providing essential building blocks for bone formation and maintenance. In this chapter, we will explore the relationship between onions and bone health, uncovering the mechanisms by which they promote skeletal resilience.

Calcium Absorption:

- Calcium is essential for bone health, providing the structural framework for bones and teeth. However, calcium absorption can be influenced by various factors, including diet and gut health.
- Onions contain prebiotic fibers, such as inulin, which serve as food for beneficial gut bacteria. These bacteria play a role in enhancing calcium absorption in the intestines, ensuring that more calcium is available for bone formation.
- By promoting healthy gut microbiota, onions support optimal calcium absorption and contribute to overall bone health.

Anti-inflammatory Effects:

- Chronic inflammation can contribute to bone loss and increase the risk of osteoporosis, a condition characterized by weakened and fragile bones.
- Onions possess anti-inflammatory properties due to their high content of antioxidants, such as quercetin and anthocyanins, which help reduce inflammation and protect against oxidative damage.
- By mitigating inflammation, onions create an environment in the body that is conducive to optimal bone health, allowing for the maintenance of strong and healthy bones.

Quercetin and Bone Density:

- Quercetin, a flavonoid antioxidant found abundantly in onions, has been studied for its potential effects on bone health.
- Research suggests that quercetin may help increase bone

density and prevent bone loss by promoting osteoblast activity, which is responsible for bone formation, and inhibiting osteoclast activity, which is responsible for bone resorption.
- By stimulating bone formation and reducing bone breakdown, quercetin may help maintain skeletal integrity and reduce the risk of osteoporosis and fractures.

Nutrient Support:

- Onions contain a variety of nutrients that are important for bone health, including vitamin C, vitamin K, and manganese.
- Vitamin C is essential for collagen synthesis, which is a key component of bone tissue.
- Vitamin K plays a role in bone metabolism and helps regulate calcium deposition in bones.
- Manganese is involved in bone formation and helps maintain bone density and strength.

Incorporating onions into a balanced diet rich in other bone-supportive nutrients, such as calcium, vitamin D, and magnesium, can help promote optimal bone health and reduce the risk of osteoporosis and fractures. Whether enjoyed raw in salads, cooked in soups and stir-fries, or caramelized in savory dishes, onions offer a delicious and nutritious way to support skeletal resilience and maintain strong and healthy bones.

Chapter 10: Onions and Blood Sugar Regulation

In an age where diabetes and insulin resistance are on the rise, onions emerge as a natural ally in the battle against unstable blood sugar levels. Packed with compounds that help regulate glucose metabolism and improve insulin sensitivity, onions offer a flavorful and versatile way to support blood sugar control and reduce the risk of diabetes-related complications. In this chapter, we will explore the relationship between onions and blood sugar regulation, uncovering the mechanisms by which these humble bulbs promote metabolic health.

Low Glycemic Index:

- Onions have a low glycemic index (GI), meaning they cause a gradual and steady increase in blood sugar levels compared to high-GI foods.
- The carbohydrates in onions are slowly digested and absorbed, leading to a more gradual release of glucose into the bloodstream and preventing spikes in blood sugar levels.
- By choosing low-GI foods like onions, individuals can better manage their blood sugar levels and reduce the risk of insulin resistance and diabetes.

Fiber Content:

- Onions are rich in dietary fiber, both soluble and insoluble, which plays a crucial role in regulating blood sugar levels.
- Soluble fiber helps slow down the absorption of glucose in the intestines, preventing rapid spikes in blood sugar levels after meals.
- Insoluble fiber adds bulk to stool and promotes digestive regularity, which can help prevent fluctuations in blood sugar levels.

Quercetin and Sulfur Compounds:

- Quercetin, a flavonoid antioxidant found abundantly in onions, has been studied for its potential effects on blood sugar regulation.
- Research suggests that quercetin may help improve insulin sensitivity and reduce fasting blood sugar levels by enhancing glucose uptake in cells and reducing insulin resistance.
- Sulfur compounds found in onions, such as allyl propyl disulfide, have also been shown to have hypoglycemic

effects, lowering blood sugar levels by stimulating insulin secretion and improving insulin sensitivity.

Anti-inflammatory Effects:

- Chronic inflammation is closely linked to insulin resistance and type 2 diabetes. Onions possess anti-inflammatory properties due to their high content of antioxidants, such as quercetin and anthocyanins.
- By reducing inflammation and oxidative stress in the body, onions help improve insulin sensitivity and support overall metabolic health.
- Including onions in a balanced diet rich in other anti-inflammatory foods can help reduce the risk of insulin resistance and diabetes-related complications.

Incorporating onions into meals as part of a balanced diet can help support blood sugar regulation and reduce the risk of diabetes. Whether enjoyed raw in salads, cooked in soups and stews, or caramelized in savory dishes, onions offer a delicious and nutritious way to promote metabolic health and enhance blood sugar control.

15

Chapter 11: Onions and Vision: Protecting Your Eyes

In a world where digital screens and environmental pollu-tants can strain our eyes, onions offer a natural solution for maintaining optimal vision and protecting eye health. Rich in antioxidants, vitamins, and minerals that support ocular function, onions serve as a flavorful and versatile addition to a vision-friendly diet. In this chapter, we will explore the relationship between onions and vision, uncovering the mechanisms by which these unassuming bulbs promote ocular wellness.

Antioxidant Protection:

- Onions are rich in antioxidants, such as quercetin, anthocyanins, and vitamin C, which help protect the eyes from oxidative damage caused by free radicals.
- Free radicals can accumulate in the eyes over time, leading to oxidative stress and contributing to age-related eye conditions such as macular degeneration and cataracts.
- By neutralizing free radicals and reducing oxidative stress, onions help preserve the health of the retina and lens, supporting clear vision and preventing vision loss.

Vitamin A:

- Onions contain vitamin A and its precursor, beta-carotene, which are essential for maintaining healthy vision.
- Vitamin A plays a crucial role in the synthesis of rhodopsin, a pigment in the retina that is necessary for low-light and color vision.
- Beta-carotene is converted into vitamin A in the body and helps protect the surface of the eye (cornea) and maintain the integrity of the mucous membranes that line the eyelids and conjunctiva.

Sulfur Compounds:

- Sulfur compounds found in onions, such as cysteine and methionine, are important for the production of glutathione, a powerful antioxidant that protects the eyes from oxidative damage.
- Glutathione plays a critical role in maintaining the transparency of the lens and preventing the formation of cataracts, a common age-related eye condition

characterized by clouding of the lens.

Anti-inflammatory Effects:

- Chronic inflammation is a contributing factor to many eye diseases, including uveitis, dry eye syndrome, and diabetic retinopathy.
- Onions possess anti-inflammatory properties due to their high content of antioxidants and sulfur compounds, which help reduce inflammation in the eyes and prevent damage to ocular tissues.
- By mitigating inflammation, onions support overall eye health and reduce the risk of inflammatory eye conditions.

Incorporating onions into a balanced diet rich in other vision-supportive nutrients, such as lutein, zeaxanthin, and omega-3 fatty acids, can help maintain optimal eye health and reduce the risk of age-related vision loss. Whether enjoyed raw in salads, cooked in soups and stews, or caramelized in savory dishes, onions offer a delicious and nutritious way to support clear vision and protect the eyes from oxidative damage.

16

Chapter 12: Onions and Skin Health

In the pursuit of radiant and youthful skin, onions may not be the first ingredient that comes to mind. However, these humble bulbs possess a remarkable array of nutrients and bioactive compounds that can nourish and rejuvenate the skin from the inside out. From promoting collagen production to combating oxidative stress, onions offer a natural and effective way to support skin health and enhance its appearance. In this chapter, we will explore the relationship between onions and skin health, uncovering the secrets behind their skin-loving properties.

Collagen Production:

- Onions contain vitamin C, which is essential for collagen synthesis, a process that helps maintain the skin's structure and elasticity.
- Collagen is a protein that provides strength and firmness to the skin, helping to reduce the appearance of wrinkles and fine lines.
- By providing the building blocks for collagen production, onions help support skin elasticity and promote a youthful complexion.

Antioxidant Protection:

- Onions are rich in antioxidants, including quercetin and anthocyanins, which help protect the skin from oxidative damage caused by free radicals.
- Free radicals can accelerate the aging process and contribute to the formation of wrinkles, age spots, and other signs of skin damage.
- By neutralizing free radicals and reducing oxidative stress, onions help preserve the skin's youthful appearance and protect against premature aging.

Anti-inflammatory Effects:

- Chronic inflammation is a common underlying factor in many skin conditions, including acne, eczema, and psoriasis.
- Onions possess anti-inflammatory properties due to their high content of antioxidants and sulfur compounds, which help reduce inflammation in the skin and alleviate symptoms of inflammatory skin conditions.

- By calming inflammation and soothing irritated skin, onions support overall skin health and promote a clear and radiant complexion.

Wound Healing:

- Onions have been used for centuries as a natural remedy for promoting wound healing and skin regeneration.
- Compounds found in onions, such as quercetin and allicin, have been shown to have antimicrobial and anti-inflammatory properties, which can help prevent infection and reduce inflammation in wounds.
- Additionally, onions contain sulfur compounds that may stimulate the production of collagen and promote the formation of new skin tissue, speeding up the healing process.

Incorporating onions into your diet and skincare routine can help nourish and protect your skin, promoting a healthy and youthful complexion. Whether enjoyed in salads, soups, or stir-fries or applied topically as part of a homemade mask or treatment, onions offer a natural and effective way to support skin health and enhance its beauty from the inside out.

17

Chapter 13: Onions: A Detoxifying Superfood

In a world filled with environmental pollutants and toxins, the body's natural detoxification processes can become over-whelmed, leading to a buildup of harmful substances that compromise health and vitality. Fortunately, onions offer a potent solution for supporting the body's detoxification pathways and promoting overall well-being. Packed with sulfur compounds, antioxidants, and fiber, onions serve as a powerful ally in the detoxification process, helping to eliminate toxins and restore balance to the body. In this chapter, we will explore the detoxifying properties of onions and their role in supporting optimal health.

Sulfur Compounds:

- Onions are rich in sulfur-containing compounds, such as cysteine and methionine, which play a crucial role in the body's detoxification pathways.
- Sulfur compounds support the production of glutathione, a powerful antioxidant that plays a central role in detoxification by neutralizing toxins and free radicals.
- Glutathione helps facilitate the removal of harmful substances from the body, including heavy metals, environmental pollutants, and metabolic waste products.

Antioxidant Protection:

- Onions contain a variety of antioxidants, including quercetin, anthocyanins, and vitamin C, which help protect cells from oxidative damage and support detoxification.
- Oxidative stress can impair detoxification pathways and contribute to the accumulation of toxins in the body. By neutralizing free radicals, antioxidants help reduce oxidative stress and support optimal detoxification.

Fiber Content:

- Onions are a good source of dietary fiber, both soluble and insoluble, which plays a key role in the detoxification process.
- Soluble fiber helps absorb toxins and waste products in the digestive tract, facilitating their elimination from the body through the stool.
- Insoluble fiber adds bulk to stool and promotes regular

bowel movements, preventing the reabsorption of toxins in the colon and supporting overall digestive health.

Liver Support:

- The liver is the body's primary detoxification organ, responsible for filtering and eliminating toxins from the bloodstream.
- Compounds found in onions, such as quercetin and sulfur compounds, have been shown to support liver function and enhance detoxification pathways.
- By promoting liver health and function, onions help ensure that toxins are efficiently processed and eliminated from the body, reducing the burden on other organs and systems.

Incorporating onions into your diet regularly can help support the body's natural detoxification processes and promote overall health and vitality. Whether enjoyed raw in salads, cooked in soups and stews, or added to smoothies and juices, onions offer a delicious and nutritious way to support detoxification and restore balance to the body.

Chapter 14: Onions and Cancer Prevention

In the fight against cancer, onions emerge as a potent ally, armed with a diverse arsenal of compounds that have been shown to inhibit tumor growth, reduce inflammation, and protect against oxidative damage. With their rich array of antioxidants, sulfur compounds, and flavonoids, onions offer a natural and effective way to support cancer prevention and promote overall well-being. In this chapter, we will explore the role of onions in cancer prevention and uncover the mechanisms by which they exert their anticancer effects.

Antioxidant Properties:

- Onions are rich in antioxidants, such as quercetin, anthocyanins, and vitamin C, which help neutralize free radicals and reduce oxidative stress in the body.
- Free radicals can damage cells and DNA, leading to mutations that can contribute to the development of cancer.
- By reducing oxidative stress and protecting against DNA damage, antioxidants in onions help lower the risk of cancer and support overall cellular health.

Anti-inflammatory Effects:

- Chronic inflammation is a key driver of cancer development, promoting tumor growth, angiogenesis, and metastasis.
- Onions possess anti-inflammatory properties due to their high content of antioxidants and sulfur compounds, which help reduce inflammation and inhibit inflammatory pathways.
- By mitigating chronic inflammation, onions help create an environment in the body that is less conducive to cancer growth and progression.

Sulfur Compounds:

- Onions contain sulfur-containing compounds, such as diallyl sulfide and allyl propyl disulfide, which have been shown to possess anticancer properties.
- These compounds have been found to inhibit the growth of cancer cells, induce apoptosis (programmed cell death), and prevent the formation of tumors in various types of cancer, including breast, colon, and prostate cancer.
- Sulfur compounds in onions may also help detoxify car-

cinogens and promote the elimination of cancer-causing substances from the body.

Quercetin and Flavonoids:

- Quercetin, a flavonoid antioxidant found abundantly in onions, has been studied for its potential anticancer effects.
- Research suggests that quercetin may help inhibit the growth and spread of cancer cells, block the formation of new blood vessels that supply tumors (angiogenesis), and enhance the effectiveness of chemotherapy and radiation therapy.
- Other flavonoids found in onions, such as anthocyanins, have also been shown to have anticancer properties, protecting against various types of cancer through their antioxidant and anti-inflammatory effects.

By incorporating onions into a balanced diet rich in other cancer-fighting foods, such as fruits, vegetables, whole grains, and lean proteins, individuals can help reduce their risk of cancer and promote overall health and well-being. Whether enjoyed raw in salads, cooked in soups and stews, or added to sandwiches and wraps, onions offer a delicious and nutritious way to support cancer prevention and unlock the secrets to a healthier future.

Chapter 15: Cooking with Onions: Tips and Techniques

Onions are not only nutritious and beneficial for health, but they also add depth, flavor, and complexity to a wide range of dishes. From soups and stews to stir-fries and salads, onions serve as a versatile culinary ingredient that can elevate the taste and texture of any meal. In this chapter, we will explore various tips and techniques for cooking with onions, unlocking their full potential in the kitchen, and enhancing their health benefits.

Selecting Onions:

- Choose onions that are firm, dry, and free of soft spots or mold. The outer skin should be papery and intact.

- Different varieties of onions offer distinct flavor profiles and are suited to different cooking methods. Experiment with yellow, white, red, and sweet onions to discover your preferences.

Preparing Onions:

- To minimize tearing when cutting onions, refrigerate them for about 30 minutes before slicing or chopping them under cold running water.
- Use a sharp knife to cut onions into uniform pieces for even cooking. Slice onions thinly for quick-cooking dishes like stir-fries or dice them finely for soups and sauces.

Cooking Techniques:

- Sautéing: Sauté sliced onions in olive oil or butter over medium heat until softened and translucent. Add sautéed onions to pasta dishes, omelets, or sandwiches for added flavor.
- Caramelizing: Slow-cook thinly sliced onions in butter or oil over low heat until golden brown and caramelized. Use caramelized onions as a topping for burgers, pizzas, or bruschetta.
- Roasting: Toss quartered onions with olive oil, salt, and pepper, then roast in the oven until tender and caramelized. Roasted onions are delicious in vegetable medleys, grain bowls, or alongside roasted meats.
- Pickling: Slice onions thinly and soak them in a mixture of vinegar, sugar, and spices to create quick-pickled onions.

Enjoy pickled onions on sandwiches, tacos, or salads for a tangy flavor boost.

Enhancing Flavor:

- Combine onions with complementary ingredients like garlic, herbs, spices, and citrus zest to enhance their flavor profile and create depth in dishes.
- Experiment with different cooking methods, such as grilling, smoking, or deep-frying, to impart unique flavors and textures to onions.

Storing Onions:

- Store onions in a cool, dry, and well-ventilated place away from direct sunlight. Avoid storing onions near potatoes, as they can cause onions to spoil more quickly.
- Once cut, store leftover onions in an airtight container in the refrigerator and use them within a few days.

By mastering the art of cooking with onions and incorporating them into a variety of dishes, you can unlock their full potential as a flavorful and nutritious ingredient. Whether used as a base for sauces and soups, a topping for pizzas and salads, or a flavorful addition to stir-fries and casseroles, onions offer endless possibilities for culinary creativity and culinary exploration. Experiment with different varieties, cooking methods, and flavor combinations to discover the many ways onions can enhance your meals and improve your health.

20

Chapter 16: Raw vs. Cooked Onions: Which is Better?

The debate between raw and cooked onions has long been a topic of discussion among food enthusiasts and health-conscious individuals alike. While both raw and cooked onions offer unique flavor profiles and nutritional benefits, understanding the differences between the two can help you make informed decisions about how to incorporate onions into your diet for maximum health benefits. In this chapter, we will explore the advantages and disadvantages of raw and cooked onions and determine which option may be better suited to your dietary preferences and health goals.

Raw Onions:

- Raw onions are pungent and crisp, with a sharp and assertive flavor that can add a punch to salads, sandwiches, and salsas.
- Raw onions contain higher levels of certain nutrients, such as vitamin C and phytonutrients like quercetin, as cooking can degrade some heat-sensitive compounds.
- Eating raw onions may provide more immediate health benefits, as the enzymes and nutrients are preserved in their natural state.
- However, raw onions can be harsh on the digestive system for some individuals, causing bloating, gas, or indigestion, especially when consumed in large quantities or by those with sensitive stomachs.

Cooked Onions:

- Cooking onions can mellow their flavor and soften their texture, making them more palatable for some people and suitable for a wider range of dishes.
- Cooked onions add depth, sweetness, and complexity to soups, stews, sauces, and stir-fries, enhancing the overall flavor profile of dishes.
- Cooking onions can increase the availability of certain nutrients, such as antioxidants and sulfur compounds, by breaking down cell walls and making them more digestible and absorbable.
- However, prolonged cooking at high temperatures can lead to nutrient loss, especially water-soluble vitamins like vitamin C. To minimize nutrient loss, consider using gentle

cooking methods like sautéing or steaming and avoiding overcooking.

Finding Balance:

- Both raw and cooked onions have their place in a healthy diet, and the best approach is to enjoy a variety of preparations to reap the full spectrum of benefits.
- Raw onions are ideal for dishes where their sharp flavor and crisp texture can shine, such as salads, sandwiches, and fresh salsas.
- Cooked onions are well-suited to dishes that benefit from their softened texture and mellow flavor, such as soups, stews, sauces, and savory baked goods.
- Experiment with different cooking methods and flavor combinations to discover the versatility of onions and find what works best for your taste preferences and dietary needs.

In conclusion, both raw and cooked onions offer distinct advantages and can be part of a healthy and balanced diet. Whether enjoyed raw or cooked, onions provide essential nutrients, antioxidants, and flavor compounds that support overall health and well-being. By incorporating a variety of onion preparations into your meals, you can unlock the full potential of these nutritious bulbs and enhance the flavor and nutritional value of your dishes.

Chapter 17: Incorporating Onions into Everyday Meals

Onions are a versatile and flavorful ingredient that can elevate the taste and nutritional value of everyday meals. From breakfast to dinner, and everything in between, there are countless ways to incorporate onions into your daily cooking routine. In this chapter, we will explore creative and delicious ways to use onions in a variety of dishes, helping you unlock the full potential of these nutritious bulbs and enhance the flavor and health benefits of your meals.

Breakfast:

- Add sautéed onions to omelets, frittatas, or scrambled eggs for a savory and satisfying start to your day.
- Top toast or bagels with caramelized onions, avocado, and a sprinkle of salt and pepper for a flavorful and nutritious breakfast option.
- Incorporate diced onions into breakfast burritos, breakfast hashes, or savory breakfast muffins for added texture and flavor.

Lunch:

- Use thinly sliced raw onions to add crunch and tang to sandwiches, wraps, and burgers. Red onions are particularly delicious in sandwiches with deli meats or grilled vegetables.
- Toss diced onions into salads for a burst of flavor and texture. Try adding them to green salads, grain salads, or pasta salads for a refreshing twist.
- Caramelize onions and use them as a topping for homemade pizzas or flatbreads, along with your favorite cheese and toppings.

Dinner:

- Start soups, stews, and chili with a base of sautéed onions, garlic, and other aromatics to build depth of flavor.
- Incorporate onions into stir-fries, curries, and rice dishes for added flavor and texture. Experiment with different onion varieties and cooking methods to create diverse flavor profiles.
- Roast or grill whole onions alongside meats or vegetables for a simple and flavorful side dish. Drizzle roasted onions

with olive oil and balsamic vinegar for an elegant and tasty accompaniment to any meal.

Snacks and Appetizers:

- Make homemade onion dip by blending caramelized onions with Greek yogurt or sour cream and seasoning with herbs and spices. Serve with fresh vegetables or whole-grain crackers for a healthy and satisfying snack.
- Stuff whole or halved onions with a mixture of breadcrumbs, cheese, herbs, and spices, then bake until tender for a delicious and impressive appetizer.
- Serve pickled onions alongside cheese and charcuterie boards for a tangy and flavorful accompaniment to your favorite snacks.

By incorporating onions into a variety of everyday meals, you can enjoy their delicious flavor and reap their numerous health benefits. Whether raw, cooked, caramelized, or pickled, onions add depth, complexity, and nutritional value to dishes, making them a versatile and essential ingredient in any kitchen. Experiment with different onion varieties, cooking techniques, and flavor combinations to discover new and exciting ways to enjoy these humble yet versatile bulbs in your everyday cooking.

Chapter 18: Onion Remedies for Common Ailments

Throughout history, onions have been valued not only as a culinary ingredient but also for their medicinal properties. Packed with beneficial compounds such as antioxidants, flavonoids, and sulfur-containing compounds, onions offer a natural and effective remedy for a variety of common ailments. In this chapter, we will explore how onions can be used to alleviate symptoms and promote healing for a range of health conditions.

Cough and Cold:

- Onion syrup: To soothe a cough and alleviate congestion,

prepare a home-made onion syrup by combining chopped onions with honey or sugar in a saucepan. Simmer the mixture over low heat until the onions are soft and the liquid has thickened into a syrup-like consistency. Strain out the onions and take a spoonful as needed to relieve cough symptoms.

- Onion poultice: For chest congestion, apply a warm onion poultice to the chest area. Grate a raw onion and wrap it in cheesecloth or a clean cloth. Place the poultice on the chest for 15-20 minutes to help loosen mucus and promote easier breathing.

Sore Throat:

- Onion gargle: For relief from a sore throat, prepare an onion gargle by boiling chopped onions in water for several minutes. Allow the mixture to cool, then strain out the onions. Gargle with the onion-infused water several times a day to reduce inflammation and soothe throat discomfort.
- Raw onion remedy: Chew on a slice of raw onion to help alleviate sore throat symptoms. The antimicrobial properties of onions can help kill bacteria and viruses that contribute to throat infections.

Insect Bites and Stings:

- Onion poultice: For relief from itching and swelling caused by insect bites and stings, apply a fresh onion poultice to the affected area. Grate or crush a raw onion and apply it directly to the bite or sting for 10-15 minutes. The natural anti-inflammatory properties of onions can help reduce swelling and irritation.

- Onion juice: Extract juice from a raw onion and apply it directly to the affected area using a cotton ball or swab. The antibacterial and antiseptic properties of onion juice can help prevent infection and promote healing.

Earache:

- Onion ear drops: To alleviate earache and ear infection symptoms, prepare homemade onion ear drops by heating chopped onions in olive oil over low heat until the onions are soft and fragrant. Allow the oil to cool, then strain out the onions. Use a dropper to administer a few drops of the onion-infused oil into the affected ear, tilting the head to allow the oil to penetrate the ear canal.

Minor Burns:

- Onion paste: For relief from minor burns and sunburn, apply a paste made from grated raw onion directly to the affected area. The natural anti-inflammatory properties of onions can help reduce pain and swelling, while the antibacterial properties can help prevent infection.

By harnessing the healing power of onions, you can effectively treat a variety of common ailments using natural and readily available ingredients. Whether used in syrups, poultices, or topical applications, onions offer a safe, affordable, and effective alternative to conventional remedies for promoting healing and alleviating symptoms. Experiment with different onion remedies to find what works best for you and enjoy the health benefits of this versatile and humble bulb.

benefits of this versatile and humble bulb.

23

Chapter 19: Onions in Traditional Medicine

For centuries, onions have held a revered place in traditional medicine systems around the world for their potent healing properties and therapeutic benefits. From ancient civilizations to modern herbalists, onions have been used to treat a wide range of ailments and promote overall health and well-being. In this chapter, we will explore the rich history of onions in traditional medicine and uncover the various ways in which they have been used to support health and vitality.

Ancient Civilizations:

- In ancient Egypt, onions were revered for their medicinal properties and were often used as a remedy for various ailments, including digestive issues, respiratory conditions, and infections. Onions were also placed in tombs as offerings to the gods and as symbols of eternal life.
- In traditional Chinese medicine (TCM), onions have been used for thousands of years to promote digestion, stimulate appetite, and relieve coughs and colds. Onions are believed to have warming properties that help dispel cold and dampness from the body.

Ayurveda:

- In Ayurvedic medicine, onions are valued for their pungent taste and heating properties, which are believed to stimulate digestion, improve circulation, and promote detoxification. Onions are often used in herbal formulations to treat respiratory conditions, digestive disorders, and inflammatory conditions.
- According to Ayurvedic principles, onions are classified as "rajasic," meaning they have stimulating and energizing qualities that can help invigorate the body and mind.

European Folk Medicine:

- In European folk medicine, onions were used as a remedy for a wide range of ailments, including colds, coughs, wounds, and infections. Onions were often applied topically as poultices or used internally as decoctions or syrups to promote healing and alleviate symptoms.
- Onions were also believed to have protective properties

against evil spirits and infectious diseases, leading to their use in rituals and as charms for warding off illness.

Modern Herbalism:

- In modern herbalism, onions are valued for their antimicrobial, anti-inflammatory, and antioxidant properties. Onions are often included in herbal formulations for respiratory health, immune support, and cardiovascular wellness.
- Onion extracts and preparations are used in herbal supplements, tinctures, and syrups to support overall health and promote healing.

While the use of onions in traditional medicine may vary across cultures and regions, their reputation as a potent healing remedy remains consistent. Whether used to alleviate coughs and colds, aid digestion, or promote overall vitality, onions continue to be valued for their therapeutic benefits and contributions to holistic health and well-being. By incorporating onions into your diet and daily routine, you can harness the healing power of this humble bulb and unlock its potential to support optimal health and vitality.

Chapter 20: Onions: A Versatile Ingredient in Beauty Regimens

In addition to their culinary and medicinal uses, onions have also found their way into beauty regimens around the world, thanks to their skin-loving properties and beneficial compounds. From promoting hair growth to improving skin tone and texture, onions offer a natural and effective way to enhance beauty and maintain healthy skin and hair. In this chapter, we will explore the various ways in which onions can be incorporated into beauty routines and unlock their potential to support radiant skin and luscious locks.

Hair Care:

- Onion juice for hair growth: Rich in sulfur compounds and antioxidants, onion juice has been used for centuries as a remedy for hair loss and promoting hair growth. Apply freshly extracted onion juice to the scalp and massage gently to stimulate blood circulation and nourish the hair follicles. Leave the juice on for 30 minutes to an hour before rinsing with water and shampooing as usual.
- Onion hair masks: Combine onion juice with other hair-friendly ingredients such as honey, coconut oil, or yogurt to create nourishing hair masks. These masks can help strengthen the hair, reduce breakage, and improve overall hair health and shine.

Skin Care:

- Onion extract for acne: Onion extract contains compounds with antimicrobial and anti-inflammatory properties that can help reduce acne breakouts and inflammation. Apply a thin layer of onion extract or onion juice to the affected areas and leave it on for 10–15 minutes before rinsing with water. Repeat daily for best results.
- Onion face masks: Mix finely grated onion with other skin-nourishing ingredients such as honey, yogurt, or aloe vera gel to create homemade face masks. These masks can help improve skin tone, reduce blemishes, and promote a clear and radiant complexion.

Nail Care:

- Onion for stronger nails: Soak fingernails or toenails in a mixture of onion juice and warm water to help strengthen weak and brittle nails. The sulfur compounds in onions can help promote nail growth and improve overall nail health.

- Onion nail soak: Slice an onion and soak nails in the juice for 10-15 minutes to help soften cuticles, strengthen nails, and prevent fungal infections.

Scalp Health:

- Onion scalp treatments: Massage onion juice or onion-infused oil into the scalp to help alleviate dandruff, dryness, and itching. The antimicrobial and anti-inflammatory properties of onions can help restore balance to the scalp and promote a healthy scalp environment.
- Onion rinses for shiny hair: Rinse hair with diluted onion juice or onion-infused water after shampooing to add shine and luster to dull and lifeless hair. The sulfur compounds in onions can help remove buildup and residue, leaving hair soft, smooth, and shiny.

Incorporating onions into your beauty regimen can help enhance your natural beauty and promote healthy skin and hair. Whether used in hair masks, face masks, or nail soaks, onions offer a natural and effective way to nourish, strengthen, and rejuvenate from head to toe. Experiment with different onion-based treatments to discover what works best for your individual needs and enjoy the beauty-enhancing benefits of this versatile and humble bulb.

Chapter 21: Growing Onions at Home: A Beginner's Guide

Growing onions at home can be a rewarding experience that allows you to enjoy fresh, flavorful bulbs while also reaping the benefits of gardening. With the right knowledge and preparation, even beginners can successfully cultivate onions in their own backyard or garden plot. In this chapter, we will provide a step-by-step guide to growing onions at home, from selecting the right variety to harvesting and storing your homegrown crop.

Choosing Onion Varieties:

- Select onion varieties that are well-suited to your climate and growing conditions. Common types of onions include yellow, white, red, and sweet onions, each with its flavor profile and culinary uses.
- Consider whether you want to grow onions from seeds, sets (small bulbs), or transplants. Sets are the easiest option for beginners, as they require less time and effort to grow than seeds.

Preparing the Soil:

- Choose a sunny location with well-draining soil for planting onions. Onions prefer loose, fertile soil with a pH of 6.0-7.5.
- Prepare the soil by loosening it with a garden fork or tiller and incorporating organic matter such as compost or aged manure to improve soil structure and fertility.

Planting Onions:

- Plant onion sets or transplants in early spring, as soon as the soil can be worked and the danger of frost has passed. Space onion sets 4-6 inches apart in rows, with rows spaced 12-18 inches apart.
- Plant onion sets or transplants with the pointed end facing up and the roots facing down. Press the sets or transplants gently into the soil so that the tops are level with the soil surface.

Caring for Onions:

- Water onions regularly, providing 1-2 inches of water per

week, especially during dry periods. Avoid over-watering, as onions are prone to rot in soggy soil.

- Mulch around onion plants with straw, shredded leaves, or grass clippings to conserve moisture, suppress weeds, and regulate soil temperature.
- Fertilize onions every 3-4 weeks with a balanced fertilizer high in nitrogen to promote healthy growth and bulb development.

Harvesting Onions:

- Onions are ready for harvest when the tops begin to yellow and flop over. To harvest, gently lift the onions from the soil with a garden fork or trowel, taking care not to damage the bulbs.
- Cure harvested onions by laying them in a single layer in a warm, dry, well-ventilated area for 1-2 weeks. Once the outer skins are dry and papery, trim the tops and roots and store the onions in a cool, dry place.

Storing Onions:

- Store cured onions in mesh bags, wire baskets, or ventilated crates in a cool, dry, and dark location such as a pantry, basement, or garage. Avoid storing onions near potatoes, as they can cause onions to spoil more quickly.
- Check stored onions regularly for signs of sprouting, rot, or decay, and remove any damaged bulbs to prevent spoilage.

By following these simple steps, you can successfully grow onions at home and enjoy a bountiful harvest of fresh, flavorful bulbs. Whether planted in a garden plot, raised bed, or container, onions are a versatile and easy-to-grow crop that can provide you with a continuous supply of nutritious and delicious bulbs for cooking and enjoying throughout the year.

26

Chapter 22: Preserving Onions for Year-round Use

While fresh onions are readily available during the growing season, preserving them allows you to enjoy their flavor and nutritional benefits year-round. From freezing and drying to pickling and fermenting, there are various methods for preserving onions that can extend their shelf life and ensure they remain a staple in your kitchen pantry. In this chapter, we will explore different techniques for preserving onions at home, allowing you to enjoy their goodness in your favorite dishes regardless of the season.

Freezing Onions:

- Chop or slice onions to your desired size and spread them out in a single layer on a baking sheet.
- Place the baking sheet in the freezer and freeze the onions until they are firm and solid.
- Transfer the frozen onions to freezer-safe bags or containers, removing as much air as possible before sealing.
- Label the bags or containers with the date and store them in the freezer for up to 6-12 months.
- Frozen onions can be used directly in cooked dishes such as soups, stews, and stir-fries without the need for thawing.

Drying Onions:

- Slice onions thinly or chop them into small pieces and spread them out in a single layer on a dehydrator tray or baking sheet.
- Dry the onions in a dehydrator or oven set to the lowest temperature until they are thoroughly dried and crisp, about 8-12 hours.
- Once dried, store the onions in an airtight container in a cool, dark place away from moisture and humidity.
- Dried onions can be rehydrated by soaking them in warm water for 15-30 minutes before using them in recipes such as soups, sauces, and casseroles.

Pickling Onions:

- Prepare a pickling brine by combining vinegar, water, sugar, and salt in a saucepan and bringing it to a boil.
- Slice onions thinly and pack them into sterilized jars along with any desired spices or flavorings.

- Pour the hot pickling brine over the onions, leaving a ½ inch of headspace at the top of the jar.
- Seal the jars with sterilized lids and process them in a water bath canner according to recommended guidelines.
- Store pickled onions in a cool, dark place for at least 1-2 weeks before consuming them to allow the flavors to develop.

Fermenting Onions:

- Slice or chop onions and pack them into a clean, sterilized jar, leaving about an inch of space at the top.
- Prepare a brine solution by dissolving salt in water (1-2 tablespoons of salt per quart of water) and pour it over the onions until they are fully submerged.
- Place a weight, such as a small plate or fermentation weight, on top of the onions to keep them submerged under the brine.
- Cover the jar with a clean cloth or fermentation lid to allow air to escape while preventing contaminants from entering.
- Ferment the onions at room temperature for 1-2 weeks, tasting them periodically until they reach the desired level of tanginess.
- Once fermented, store the onions in the refrigerator where they will continue to ferment slowly over time.

By preserving onions using these methods, you can ensure a steady supply of this versatile ingredient for year-round use in your favorite recipes. Whether frozen, dried, pickled, or fermented, preserved onions retain their flavor and nutritional value, allowing you to enjoy the goodness of onions in all seasons. Experiment with different preservation techniques and discover new ways to incorporate onions into your culinary creations for delicious and nutritious meals anytime, anywhere.

27

Chapter 23: Exploring the Cultural Significance of Onions

Throughout history, onions have played a significant role in the culinary traditions, folklore, and cultural practices of diverse societies around the world. From ancient civilizations to modern-day cultures, onions have been revered for their versatility, flavor, and nutritional value, as well as their symbolism and significance in various cultural contexts. In this chapter, we will explore the cultural significance of onions in different regions and societies, shedding light on the rich tapestry of stories, traditions, and beliefs associated with this humble yet revered vegetable.

Ancient Egypt:

- In ancient Egypt, onions were highly prized for their medicinal properties and were used as a remedy for various ailments, including digestive issues, respiratory conditions, and infections. Onions were also associated with fertility, rebirth, and eternal life, leading to their inclusion in burial rituals and offerings to the gods.
- The ancient Egyptians believed that onions symbolized protection and were used as amulets to ward off evil spirits and promote health and well-being.

Mediterranean:

- In Mediterranean cuisine, onions are a staple ingredient that forms the foundation of many dishes, from soups and stews to salads and sauces. Onions are often caramelized or sautéed to add depth and sweetness to savory dishes, and their pungent flavor is celebrated in traditional recipes such as French onion soup and Greek spanakopita.
- In Mediterranean folklore, onions are associated with love, fertility, and prosperity, and are often used in rituals and celebrations to bring good fortune and ward off negative energy.

Asia:

- In Asian cultures, onions are valued for their medicinal properties and are used in traditional medicine to treat a variety of health conditions, including colds, coughs, and digestive disorders. Onions are also incorporated into

culinary dishes such as stir-fries, curries, and noodle dishes, where they add flavor, texture, and nutritional value.
- In Chinese folklore, onions are associated with protection, purification, and prosperity, and are often included in rituals and ceremonies to bring luck and ward off evil spirits.

Europe:

- In European folklore, onions are believed to have protective properties and were used as charms and talismans to ward off illness, evil spirits, and negative energy. Onions were also associated with love, fertility, and prosperity, and were often included in wedding ceremonies and fertility rituals.
- In European cuisine, onions are a versatile ingredient that is used in a wide range of dishes, from classic French onion soup to Italian pasta sauces and Spanish omelets. Onions are often celebrated for their ability to add depth, flavor, and complexity to savory dishes, and are prized for their culinary versatility.

Middle East:

- In Middle Eastern cuisine, onions are a fundamental ingredient that forms the basis of many traditional dishes, such as kebabs, tagines, and mezze spreads. Onions are often caramelized, grilled, or pickled to enhance their flavor and add depth to savory dishes.
- In Middle Eastern folklore, onions are associated with strength, protection, and purification, and are often used in rituals and ceremonies to ward off negative energy and bring good fortune.

From ancient times to the present day, onions have held a special place in the hearts and minds of people around the world, serving as a symbol of nourishment, healing, and cultural identity. Whether used in cooking, medicine, or folklore, onions continue to play a vital role in shaping the traditions and beliefs of diverse cultures, enriching our lives with their flavor, symbolism, and significance.

28

Chapter 24: Myths and Misconceptions About Onions

Despite their long history of culinary and medicinal use, onions have often been the subject of myths and misconceptions. From exaggerated health claims to unfounded fears, these misconceptions can obscure the true value and potential of onions as a nutritious and versatile ingredient. In this chapter, we will debunk some of the most common myths and misconceptions about onions, allowing you to separate fact from fiction and fully appreciate the benefits of incorporating onions into your diet and lifestyle.

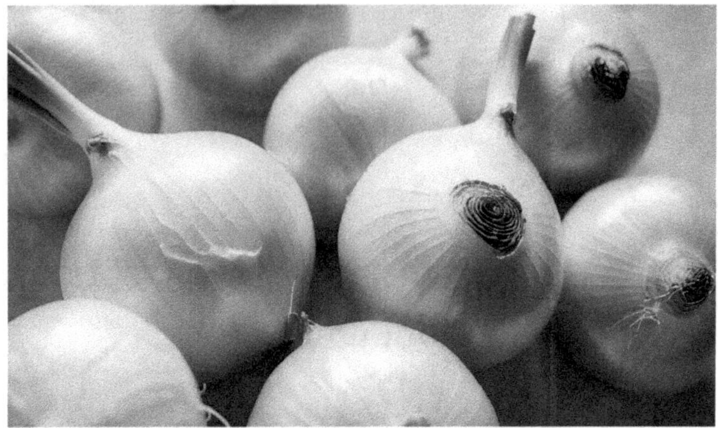

Myth: Onions are unhealthy because they make you cry when you chop them.

Fact: While chopping onions can cause tears due to the release of sulfur compounds, onions themselves are highly nutritious and beneficial for health. They are rich in antioxidants, vitamins, and minerals that support overall well-being, including heart health, immune function, and digestive wellness. The tears induced by chopping onions are a temporary inconvenience and do not diminish the nutritional value of the vegetable.

Myth: Onions are bad for digestion and can cause stomach upset.

Fact: Onions are a rich source of dietary fiber, which can promote digestive health by supporting regular bowel movements and preventing constipation. While some individuals may experience digestive discomfort from onions, such as gas or bloating, this is typically due to their high fructan content, which can be problematic for those with irritable bowel syndrome (IBS) or fructose malabsorption. For most people, onions are well-tolerated and can be enjoyed as part of a balanced diet.

Myth: Onions are high in sugar and should be avoided by people with diabetes.

Fact: While onions do contain natural sugars, they are also low in calories and have a low glycemic index, meaning they have a minimal impact on blood sugar levels when consumed in moderation. Onions are rich in fiber and antioxidants, which can help regulate blood sugar levels and improve insulin sensitivity. When included as part of a balanced meal, onions can be a nutritious addition to the diet of individuals with diabetes.

Myth: Onions are a cure-all for various health conditions.

Fact: While onions have been valued for their medicinal properties for centuries, they are not a miracle cure for all ailments. While onions contain beneficial compounds such as antioxidants and anti-inflammatory agents, they should be consumed as part of a balanced diet and healthy lifestyle, rather than relied upon as a sole remedy for health issues. While onions can certainly contribute to overall health and well-being, they should be viewed as one component of a holistic approach to wellness.

Myth: Red onions are spicier and more pungent than other varieties.

Fact: The flavor and pungency of onions are influenced by a variety of factors, including their sulfur content, growing conditions, and storage methods, rather than their color. While red onions do tend to have a slightly milder flavor compared to white or yellow onions, individual preferences for onion flavor can vary widely. Regardless of color, onions can be enjoyed in a variety of dishes and culinary applications to enhance flavor and nutritional value.

By dispelling these myths and misconceptions, we can better appreciate the true value and potential of onions as a nutritious and versatile ingredient that can enhance our health and well-being. By incorporating onions into our diet and lifestyle in moderation, we can enjoy their delicious flavor, culinary versatility, and numerous health benefits without falling prey to unfounded fears or misconceptions.

29

Chapter 25: Embracing Onions for a Healthier Life

In the journey to optimal health and well-being, embracing the humble onion can be a simple yet powerful step. With its rich array of nutrients, versatile culinary applications, and centuries-old tradition of medicinal use, the onion offers a wealth of benefits for the body, mind, and spirit. In this final chapter, we will explore how incorporating onions into your diet and lifestyle can help you unlock the secrets to a healthier, happier life.

Nutritional Powerhouse:

- Onions are a nutritional powerhouse, packed with vitamins, minerals, and antioxidants that support overall health and vitality. From immune-boosting vitamin C to bone-strengthening calcium and heart-healthy potassium, onions offer a bounty of essential nutrients that nourish the body from the inside out.

Culinary Versatility:

- With their unique flavor profile and versatile texture, onions are a culinary staple in cuisines around the world. Whether raw, cooked, caramelized, or pickled, onions add depth, complexity, and nutritional value to a wide range of dishes, from soups and salads to stir-fries and sandwiches. By incorporating onions into your favorite recipes, you can elevate the taste and nutritional quality of your meals while enjoying the health benefits of this humble bulb.

Medicinal Benefits:

- Beyond their culinary uses, onions have a long history of medicinal use in traditional healing systems around the world. Rich in antioxidants, anti-inflammatory compounds, and antimicrobial agents, onions offer a natural and effective remedy for a variety of health conditions, including colds, coughs, digestive issues, and skin ailments. By harnessing the healing power of onions, you can support your body's natural ability to heal and thrive.

Holistic Wellness:

- Embracing onions for a healthier life goes beyond just their nutritional and medicinal benefits—it's about embracing a holistic approach to wellness that nourishes the body, mind, and spirit. By cultivating a deeper connection with food and the natural world, you can foster a sense of balance, harmony, and vitality that extends to every aspect of your life.

Simple Pleasures:

- Finally, embracing onions for a healthier life is about appreciating the simple pleasures that they bring to our daily lives. From the aroma of onions sizzling in a pan to the satisfaction of biting into a crisp, flavorful slice, onions offer moments of joy and nourishment that remind us to savor the present moment and celebrate the abundance of nature's gifts.

In conclusion, onions are more than just a humble vegetable—they are a source of nourishment, healing, and joy that can enrich our lives in countless ways. By embracing onions for a healthier life, you can tap into their transformative power and unlock the secrets to a life filled with vitality, wellness, and abundance. So go ahead, savor the flavor, reap the benefits, and let onions be your guide on the journey to a healthier, happier you.

30

Chapter 30

www.ingramcontent.com/pod-product-compliance
Lightning Source LLC
Chambersburg PA
CBHW050834260726
48660CB00006B/2226